Soumia Benbernou
Nabil Ghomari
Rabeh Kouadria

Diagnosis and management of post-operative peritonitis

Soumia Benbernou
Nabil Ghomari
Rabeh Kouadria

Diagnosis and management of post-operative peritonitis

Postoperative peritonitis

ScienciaScripts

Imprint

Any brand names and product names mentioned in this book are subject to trademark, brand or patent protection and are trademarks or registered trademarks of their respective holders. The use of brand names, product names, common names, trade names, product descriptions etc. even without a particular marking in this work is in no way to be construed to mean that such names may be regarded as unrestricted in respect of trademark and brand protection legislation and could thus be used by anyone.

Cover image: www.ingimage.com

This book is a translation from the original published under ISBN 978-620-6-71056-1.

Publisher:
Sciencia Scripts
is a trademark of
Dodo Books Indian Ocean Ltd. and OmniScriptum S.R.L publishing group

120 High Road, East Finchley, London, N2 9ED, United Kingdom
Str. Armeneasca 28/1, office 1, Chisinau MD-2012, Republic of Moldova, Europe
Printed at: see last page
ISBN: 978-620-7-61670-1

Copyright © Soumia Benbernou, Nabil Ghomari, Rabeh Kouadria
Copyright © 2024 Dodo Books Indian Ocean Ltd. and OmniScriptum S.R.L publishing group

DIAGNOSIS AND MANAGEMENT OF POST-OPERATIVE PERITONITIS

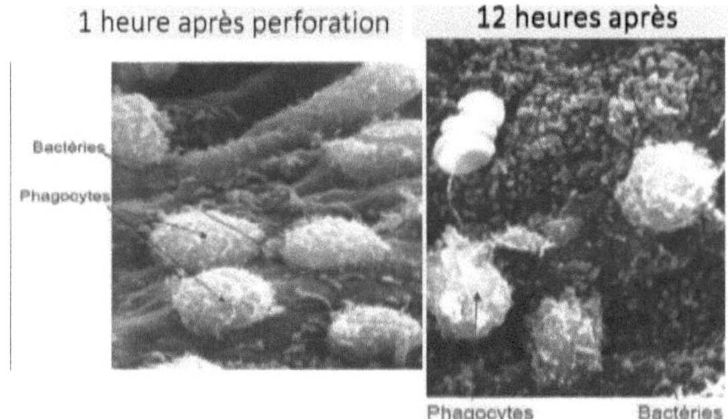

SOUMIA BENBERNOU - NABIL GHOMARI - RABEH KOUADRIA

"First and foremost, we thank God, the Almighty, for giving uśthe strength to survive, as well as the boldness to overcome all difficulties.
To you be praise, glory, honour and every blessing".

CONTENTS

I. INTRODUCTION AND ISSUES

Post-operative peritonitis (PPO) is the most feared complication following abdomino-pelvic surgery, particularly digestive surgery. The principle of their management is based on early diagnosis, optimal surgical control of the infectious source, appropriate antibiotic therapy and management of organ failure.The patient's prognosis can be complicated by the multi-resistant nature of the germs involved, risking inadequate antibiotic therapy, and by the patient's previous comorbidities, leading to the development of sepsis and organ failure. All these factors explain the high mortality rate following peritonitis. However, few studies have looked at the risk factors for mortality. The main aim of this study was to determine the epidemiological and clinical characteristics of post-operative peritonitis in patients hospitalised in the intensive care unit, as well as to define the incidence of occurrence of PPO and their evolution.

❖ Issues and objectives of the study

- To determine the epidemiological and clinical characteristics of PPO hospitalised in the intensive care unit of the Mostaganem University Hospital.

- Defining the incidence of PPO

- Keeping abreast of developments in PPOs

"

II. LITERATURE ON OPP 1-DEFINITION

Post-operative peritonitis (PPO) is secondary and tertiary nosocomial peritonitis following surgery. They complicate between 1.5 and 3.5% of laparotomies. The etiologies are dominated by anastomotic disunion. Hospital mortality remains above 25%. Untreated postoperative peritonitis is rapidly accompanied by organ failure. The incidence of multi-resistant bacteria is higher than in community-acquired peritonitis.

2- Diagnosis: Is often difficult.

A- General signs: general condition rapidly altered, the patient is frozen, has a drawn face with dry lips and pinched wings of the nose. This is the classic peritoneal facies.

Fever: either absent or present at 39 to 40°c, sometimes replaced by hypothermia with a poor prognosis.

B- Physical signs such as pain or meteorism **are** often difficult to interpret in a recently operated patient.

Sometimes there is an abnormal flow through a drainage orifice, an increase in the volume of digestive aspiration or multi-visceral failure, all of which have a poor prognosis.

C- Biological disturbances: early hyponatraemia, hypokalaemia, increased uraemia and increased white blood cell counts.

NB: Post-operative peritonitis should be considered whenever the post-operative course is disturbed (in the presence of any post-operative complication).

3- Additional examinations

Morphological examinations, particularly CT scans with digestive and vascular opacification, are essential to establish the diagnosis. Surgical management, supported by intensive care, must be carried out as early as possible before the onset of multi-visceral failure, which has a poor prognosis.

4- Diagnosis of severity

The severity of acute peritonitis may depend on the terrain, the patient's clinical condition at the time of diagnosis, the biological work-up, the aetiological diagnosis and even the speed with which therapeutic measures are implemented.

The seriousness of the situation can be summarised as follows:

✓ Terrain (diabetes, coronary artery disease, immunodepression, failure to thrive, etc.) of a system...)

✓ Clinical elements:

Shock Respiratory distress
Neurological distress

✓ Biological elements :

Renal insufficiency (disturbance of renal function urea and creatininemia)
Ionic disorders Respiratory failure Metabolic acidosis
Haemostasis disorders (decreased PT, thrombocytopenia)

✓ Aetiological elements: Stercoral peritonitis

Peritonitis due to neoplastic complications

5- Pathophysiology

A local cause involving chemical or sceptic inoculation of an abdominal viscera. This inoculation can occur either by perforation or diffusion.

These are polymicrobial infections linked to pathogenic intestinal flora:

Enterobacteria (Escherichia coli) and **anaerobes**

(Bacteroidesfragilis) whose virulence is enhanced by an aero-anaerobic synergy.

The following are due :

● Or to the disunion of a digestive anastomosis facilitated by a surgical technique.

● Or superinfection of a collection of blood or lymph favoured by a lack of haemostasis or inadequate abdominal drainage.

The most common type is a medium or low digestive perforation, ileal or colonic. Through the perforation flows faecal or ileal fluid, which contains a high concentration of aerobic and anaerobic germs.

Intense peritoneal inflammation leads to fluid sequestration, with the appearance of a 3rd sector, paralytic ileus and hypovolaemia.

These germs contain endotoxins which enter the general circulation through the peritoneal serosa, causing peripheral vasodilatation, reduced venous return and myocardial failure, all of which contribute to the onset of septic shock.

Manifestations secondary to peritonitis :

PPOs affect the body's major functions:

1. Circulatory failure: due to

• Hypovolaemia: due to the 3ème sector and aggravated by vomiting.

• The action of endotoxins, which alter peripheral resistance.

• Myocardial incompetence.

This circulatory failure leads to a severe state of shock which is initially reversible with treatment, but rapidly becomes irreversible.

2. Acute renal failure :

-Oliguric or anuric ARF is directly linked to hypovolaemia, is most often functional and is related to cortical renal ischaemia with a drop in glomerular filtration.

-Infectious shock can cause organic ARF due to tubulointerstitial nephropathy.

3. Acute respiratory failure :

Acute respiratory failure initially results from a reduction in ventilation through direct mechanical action: distension of the abdomen, contracture of the wall and reduced diaphragmatic clearance. Secondly, hypoxia is aggravated by metabolic acidosis, while septic peritonitis increases tissue oxygen requirements.

4. Acute metabolic failure :

Metabolic acidosis and hyperlactataemia occur as a result of reduced tissue perfusion and oxygenation. Coagulation is impaired, with a fall in prothrombin complex factors (II, V, VII, X), fibrin levels and platelet numbers.

5. Hepatic failure: results in

• Impaired coagulation function.

• Mixed variable jaundice with cholestasis and cytolysis.

6. Neurological disorders :

Frequent obnubilation and delirium linked to hypoxia, hypovolaemia and the action of bacterial toxins on the brain.

6- Treatment :

<u>A.</u> Goals :

-Correct the disorders and general consequences of peritonitis as quickly as possible.
-Treating peritonitis

- Eliminate the cause of the peritonitis.

<u>B.</u> Resources

1. Medical treatment :

The aim is to rapidly correct fluid and electrolyte disorders, combat the systemic spread of the infection with antibiotic therapy (as appropriate as possible) and control visceral failure. This medical treatment must be energetic and of short duration in order to bring to the operating theatre a balanced patient who can undergo general anaesthesia in the best possible conditions, and it must be continued during and after the operation.

▪ **Correction of hydro-electrolyte disorders:** By inserting a venous line, a gastric tube for digestive suction, and a bladder catheter to collect hourly diuresis. If there is cardiac disease or if massive filling is planned, a central venous catheter must be inserted to measurement of CVP. The rate of infusion should be adjusted according to the extent of hydroelectrolytic losses, as assessed clinically (dry mucous membranes, skin folds, etc.) and biologically (urea, haematocrit, ionogram, etc.).

▪ **Respiratory failure** justifies nasotracheal intubation and ventilatory assistance.

▪ **Antibiotic therapy :**

It must be massive, administered by the IV route and active on the germs usually involved; gram (-) and anaerobic germs should be avoided. Either a combination of a beta-lactam, an aminoglycoside and metronidazole, or amoxicillin-clavulanic acid and an aminoglycoside will be given. This antibiotic therapy will then be adapted to the results of intraoperative samples, to improve the effectiveness of the treatment.

2. Surgical treatment :

The aim of surgical treatment is to remove the cause of septic contamination and clean the peritoneal cavity.

➜ Generalised peritonitis: recovery by laparotomy, cleansing peritoneal +/-stomies and drainage. No digestive suture.

➜ Douglas abscess: drainage either by posterior colpotomy in women, or rectotomy in men or children.

➜ Subphrenic abscess: percutaneous or surgical drainage.

III. MATERIAL AND METHOD

1. Type of study

This is a retrospective descriptive study of cases with postoperative peritonitis that occurred between 10 September 2022 and 11 February 2023 (05 months) at the Mostaganem University Hospital.

2. Population studied

Patients operated on for digestive surgery at Mostaganem University Hospital and managed postoperatively in the Intensive Care Unit.

3. Inclusion and exclusion criteria

● **Inclusion criteria :**

- All patients diagnosed with postoperative peritonitis within 05 months.
- Over 15 years of age.

● **Exclusion criteria :**

- All patients with a diagnosis that does not correspond to the definition of postoperative peritonitis.
- Under 15 years of age.

4. Procedure for collecting data

● Work in progress

The patient files to be collected were identified on the databases of the Intensive Care Unit, the Operating Theatre and the General Surgery Department of the Mostaganem University Hospital.

Pre-, intra- and postoperative clinical data from the first and second operations, with follow-up in the intensive care unit (from the diagnosis of peritonitis) or until the patient's death or discharge, were collected in an observation notebook shown in **Tables 01; 02; 04 and 08**.

The data collected were :

-Demographics: age, gender, medical history (heart disease, hypertension, diabetes), smoking and obesity.

-Surgical: initial pathology, initial operation, duration of treatment

surgery.

• Clinical diagnosis: time to onset of first postoperative symptoms, signs of onset (shock, abdominal pain, respiratory distress, neurological distress, other or combination of several symptoms).
-Biological diagnosis (day of diagnosis): white blood cell count, CRP.
-Surgical revision: time between discovery and revision, cause of

PPO.

• Post-operative therapies: ATB administered

• The final outcome is linked to the episode of PPO: death or discharge from hospital. intensive care unit.

5. Analysis Statistics

Quantitative data were expressed as the mean according to their normal or asymmetric distribution. Qualitative data were expressed as numbers and percentages. Statistical analysis will be carried out using SPSS software (IBM SPSS Statistics for Windows).

IV. RESULTS

I. Descriptive study of data

1. Demographic data and comorbidities

Reported in the first table.

Patient name	Gender of patient	Age	HT A	Diabetes	Cardiopathy	Taba c	Obesity
B	H	62	Yes	No	HVG	Yes	Yes
B	H	58	No	No	No	Yes	No
G	F	71	Yes	Type 2	No	No	No
O	H	71	Yes	Type 1	ACFA	No	Yes
M	F	75	No	No	No	No	No
B	H	52	Yes	No	No	No	No
B	F	79	No	No	No	No	No
B	F	21	No	No	No	No	Yes
G	H	63	Yes	No	No	Yes	Yes
B	H	67	No	No	No	No	No
B	H	60	No	No	No	No	No
C	F	68	Yes	Yes	Yes	No	Yes

Table 01: Data on patients admitted to the intensive care unit at Mostaganem University Hospital from 10 September 2022 to 11 February 2023 (05 months): age, history.

Patients ranged in age from 21 to 79 years, with a mean age of From 62.25 years old. The male/female sex ratio was 1.4, i.e. 07 men to 5 women. Shown in Figure 01.

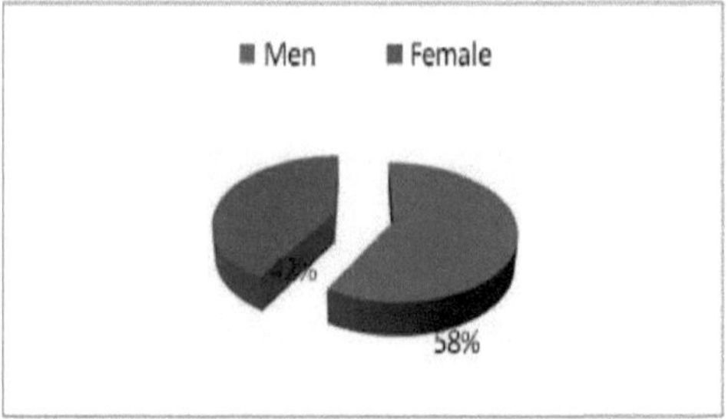

Figure 01: Sex distribution of patients hospitalised in the intensive care unit at Mostaganem University Hospital from 10 September 2022 to 11 February 2023 (05 months).

The main co-morbidities found in our patients are HTA (50%), obesity (41.7%), diabetes and heart disease (25%). As for smoking, 25% of our patients were smokers. Shown in Figures 02, 03, 04, 05 and 06.

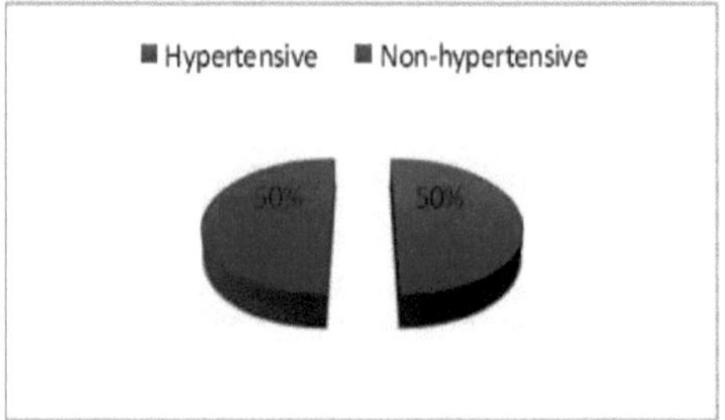

Figure 02: Percentage of hypertensive patients hospitalised in the intensive care unit at Mostaganem University Hospital from 10 September 2022 to 11 February 2023.

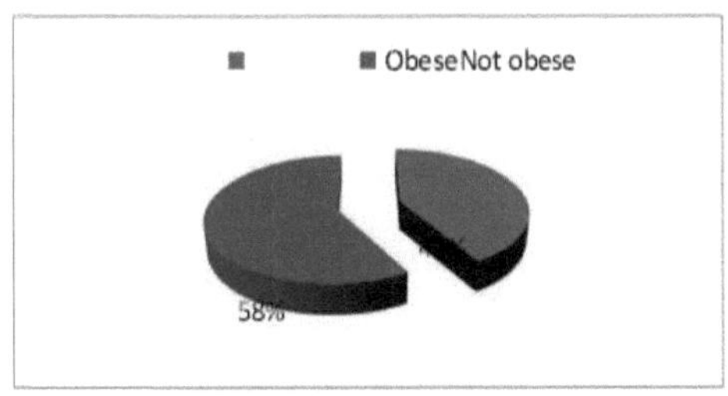

Figure 03: Percentage of obese patients hospitalised in the intensive care unit at Mostaganem University Hospital from 10 September 2022 to 11 February 2023.

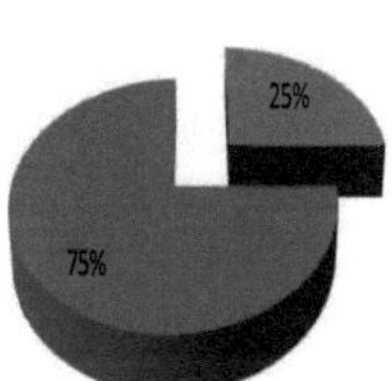

Figure 04: Percentage of diabetic patients hospitalised in the intensive care unit at Mostaganem University Hospital from 10 September 2022 to 11 February 2023.

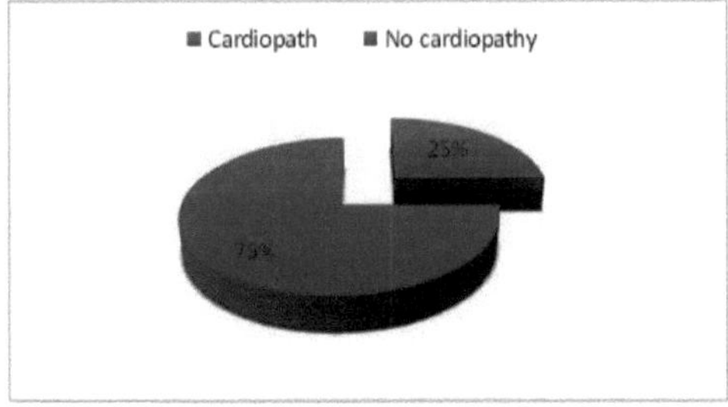

Figure 05: Percentage of patients with heart disease admitted to the intensive care unit at Mostaganem University Hospital from 10 September 2022 to 11 February 2023

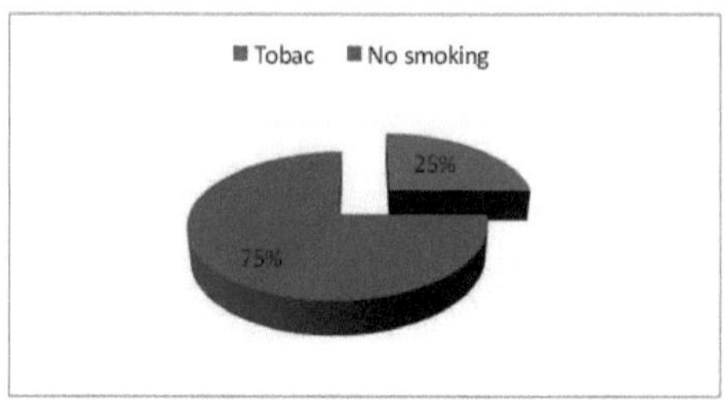

Figure 06: Percentage of smoking patients hospitalised in the intensive care unit at Mostaganem University Hospital from 10 September 2022 to 11 February 2023.

2. Clinical and biological data at the time of diagnosis of PPO
Reported in table 02.

Patient name	PPO Discovery Day	Signs of discovery (abdominal pain; shock; DR; DN)	The time between discovery and return to the operating theatre	CRP and GB biology
B	J5	Abdominal pain	01 day	300 /1 7700
B	J3	The state of shock	02 days	122 / 8400
G	J7	Shock and DR and DN	not included (IDM)	384 / 24870
O	J4	The state of shock and abdominal pain	02 days	144 / 9500
M	J3	The state of shock	00 days	200 / 25500
B	J21	Abdominal pain	15 days	102 / 15780
B	J10	Abdominal pain	04 days	200 / 11600
B	J3	The state of shock	01 day	150 / 6630
G	J4	Abdominal pain, fever and vomiting	00 days	95.5 / 12000
B	J17	Abdominal pain	03 days	120 / 16500
B	J5	Abdominal pain and state of shock	00 days	100/ 10800
C	J0	The state of shock	00 days	100 / 12000

Table 02: Clinical and paraclinical data of patients hospitalised in the intensive care unit of Mostaganem University Hospital from 10 September 2022 to 11 February 2023.

The average time to onset of symptoms after the initial surgery was 4.67 days, with extremes of 1 to 10 days, the highest percentage being 03 days. The signs of discovery varied between abdominal pain (34%) and shock (33%), while their association was 25%. The other signs were 8%, as shown in Figure 07 and Table 03.

VariablesValue (n = 12)	1- The clinic
Digestive symptoms of PPO	Abdominal pain4 (34%)
Other symptoms Fever	01 (08%)
Shock on resumption	04 (33%)
Neurological distress	00
Respiratory distress	00
Combination of several symptoms	03 (25%)
2- Biology	
CRP at recovery (mg/l) ** (n = 12 cases)	159.7 [95.5 ; 384]
White blood cell count14	14 106.66 [6 630 ; 25 500]

Table 03: Interpretation of clinical and paraclinical data at the time of diagnosis of PPO in patients hospitalised in the intensive care unit of Mostaganem University Hospital from 10 September 2022 to 11 February 2023.

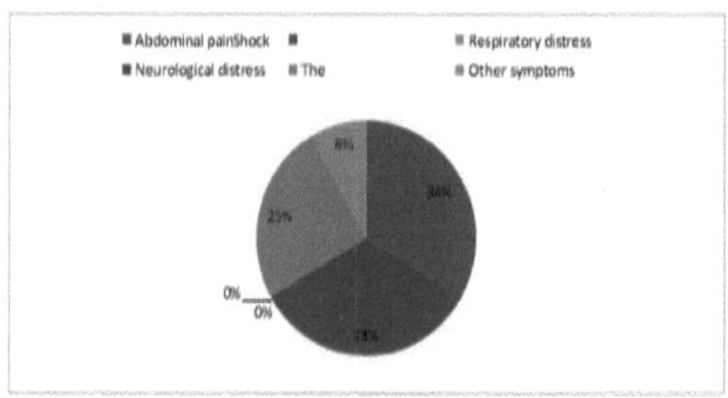

Figure 07: Percentage distribution of clinical signs of discovery of OPP in patients hospitalised in the intensive care unit at Mostaganem University Hospital from 10 September 2022 to 11 February 2023.

Empirical antibiotic therapy is based on monotherapy at 8%, dual therapy at 50% and triple therapy at 42%. antibiotics administered are: Tienam; Flagyl; Claforan; Amykacin; Gentamycin; Ciprofloxacin. Shown in Figure 08.

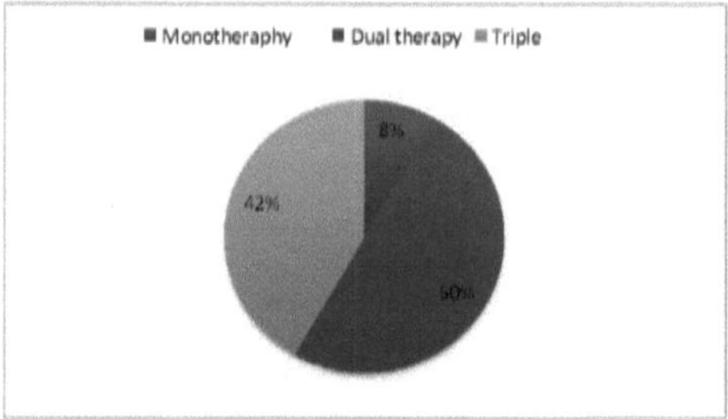

Figure 08: Percentage of antibiotic therapy used in the management of PPO in patients hospitalised in the intensive care unit of Mostaganem University Hospital from 10 September 2022 to 11 February 2023.

3. Data surgical

Reported in table 04.

Patient name	Initial pathology	Initial intervention	Initial intervention time
B	Colon neoplasia	Left hemi-colectomy	02 h
		+ colorectal anastomosis	
B	Gastric neoplasia	Total gastrectomy + anastomosis with Y-shaped loop	03 h
G	Gastric neoplasia	Total gastrectomy + anastomosis with Y-shaped loop	04h
O	Neoplasia of the recto-sigmoid hinge	Tumour resection + colorectal anastomosis	02 h
M	Bile duct neoplasia	External bypass of the bile (The MEP of a drain)	02h
B	Vesicular lithiasis	cholecystectomy under laparoscopy	01 h
B	Neoplasia of the cecum and ascending colon	Tumour resection + colorectal anastomosis	02 h
B	HTIC	Ventriculo-peritoneal shunt	
G	Colon neoplasia (loop sigmoidal)	Left hemi-colectomy + colostomy	03h
B	Neoplasia of the rectum	Colostomy and restoration of ontinuity	3h
B	Sigmoid volvulus	Colostomy and restoration of continuity	
C	LVBP	ERCP	2h

Table 04: Data on the initial surgical pathology of patients operated on at Mostaganem University Hospital from 10 September 2022 to 11 February 2023.

Patients operated on for digestive surgery (67% carcinological pathology, 17% biliary pathology, 8% for occlusive pathology and HTIC) at the CHU of Mostaganem and cared for post-operatively in the Intensive Care Unit, which is shown in the following figure 09.

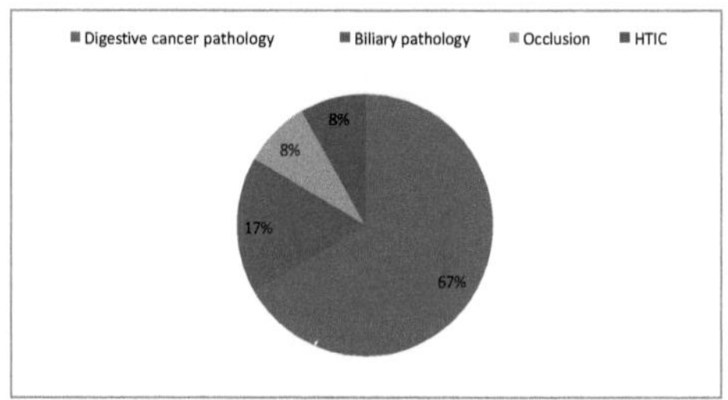

Figure 09: Percentage distribution of initial pathology of patients operated on at Mostaganem University Hospital from 10 September 2022 to 11 February 2023.

As regards the aspects relating to the surgical resumption, on average the discovery day is 4.67 days with a minimum of 1 and a maximum of 10, 25% of which are discovered on the 03rd day, as shown in Table 05.

Frequen ce			Percentage age
Vali de	Less than 3 days	1	8,3
	3 days	3	25,0
	4 days	2	16,7
	5 days	2	16,7
	7 days	1	8,3
	10 days	1	8,3
	More than 10 days	2	16,7
	Total	12	100,0

Table 05: The OPP Discovery Day.

The average time between discovery and recovery was 3.33 days, with a minimum of 1 day and a maximum of 06 days. Of these, 33.3% were taken back on the same day as the discovery, as shown in table 06.

Frequen ce			Percentage
Vali de	Not included	1	8,3
	0 day	4	33,3
	1 day	2	16,7
	2 days	2	16,7
	3 days	1	8,3
	More than 3 days	2	16,7
	Total	12	100,0

Table 06: Time between discovery and recovery in the operating theatre.

The main cause of peritonitis was a loose anastomosis (58.3%), as shown in Table 07.Frequency			Pource ntage
Val ide	Releasing the anastomosis	7	58,3
	Disinsertion of drain	1	8,3
	Aberrant channel	1	8,3
	Perforation of an organ	2	16,7
	Suture loosening	1	8,3
Total		12	100,0

Table 07: Causes of PPO.

4. Post-operative period and outcome of patients

Shown in Table 08.

Patient name	The cause of PPO	Antibiotic therapy used	The evolution
B	Anastomosis release	Tienam; Amikacin; Cancidaz	Outgoing
B	Anastomosis release	Tienam; Flagyl; Amikacin	Deceased
G	Anastomosis release	Cefacidal	Deceased
O	Anastomosis release	Tienam; Gentamycin	Deceased
M	Disinsertion of the drain	Tienam; Flagyl	Deceased
B	Aberrant channel	Tenam; Ciprolon	deceased
B	Anastomosis release	Claforon; Flagyl	Outgoing e
B	Greek perforation	Tienam; Claforan; Flagyl	Outgoing e
G	Lower segment suture loosening	Tienam; Flagyl; Ciprol; Amikacin	Deceased
B	Anastomosis release	Claforon; Flagyl; Gentamycune	Outgoing
B	Anastomosis release	Claforon; Flagyl	Deceased
C	Duodenal perforation	Teinam; Flagyl	Deceased

Table 08: Causes; Treatment; Evolution of PPO of patients hospitalised in the intensive care unit at Mostaganem University Hospital from 10 September 2022 to 11 February 2023.

Empirical antibiotic prescriptions in accordance with the department's protocols were maintained in 08 cases and modified in 04 cases as part of a therapeutic escalation. In terms of outcome, there were 08 deaths, i.e. 66.7% of the patients shown. in Figure 10.

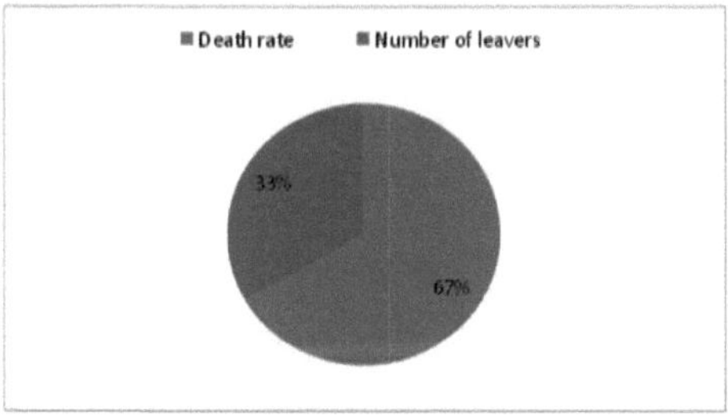

Figure 10: Mortality rate of PPO patients hospitalised in the intensive care unit of Mostaganem University Hospital from 10 September 2022 to 11 February 2023.

2Analytical study

The comparison of the different parameters (demographic; pre-, intra- and postoperative) between the two groups who left (n = 04) and died (n = 08) is presented in Tables 09, 10, 11, 12 and 13. In the analysis, the comparison of epidemiological variables (age, sex, pathological history) :

-The mean age at onset of PPO was higher in deceased patients (64.75 vs 57.25 years) than in patients discharged from the intensive care unit.

-Sex: the occurrence of PPO was higher in males in patients who died than in patients discharged from the intensive care unit, where the sex ratio was 1.

-Pathological history: occurrence of PPO (hypertension, diabetes, obesity, heart disease, smoking) was higher in patients who died than in patients discharged from the intensive care unit. Clinical and therapeutic data: Patients who died (37.5% vs. 25%) had a higher incidence of shock on recovery than patients discharged from the intensive care unit.The incidence of abdominal pain on recovery was higher in patients discharged from the ICU (7% vs. 12.5%), and this difference was statistically significant.There were statistically significant differences in the surgical data, in particular the origin of the peritonitis (neoplastic pathology predominated in the 2 groups of patients compared with the other pathologies) and the cause of the PPO (or release of the anastomosis was the most frequent cause of PPO whatever the patients who died or were discharged (3/1S; 4/1D) compared with the other causes of PPO). With regard to the antibiotic therapy used : In the case of patients who died, the use of dual therapy was higher at 62.5%, whereas in the group of patients who were discharged, the use of triple therapy was higher at 75%.

Features	Leavers (n = 04)	Deceased (n =08)
Age	57.25 [21 ; 79]	64.75 [52 ; 75]
Type		
Female Male	2 (50%) 2 (50%)	3 (37.5%) 5 (62.5%)
HTA		
Yes No	1 (25%) 3 (75%)	5 (62.5%) 3 (37.5%)
Diabetes		
Yes No	0 (00%) 4 (100%)	3 (37.5%) 5 (62.5%)
Obesity		
Yes	2 (50%)	3 (37,5%)
No	2 (50%)	5 (62,5%)
Heart disease		
Yes No	1 (25) 3 (75)	2 (25) 6 (75)
Smoking		
Yes No	1 (25) 3 (75)	2 (25) 6 (75)

Table 09: Comparison of preoperative data between the Discharged

and Deceased groups (n=12)

Features	Leavers (n = 04)	Deceased (n = 08)
1- THE CLINIC		
Digestive symptoms of OPP Abdominal pain	3 (75%)	1 (12.5%)
Other symptoms Fever	0 (00%)	1 (12.5%)
Shock on resumption	1 (25%)	3 (37.5%)
Neurological distress	0 (00%)	0 (00%)
Respiratory distress	0 (00%)	0 (00%)
Combination of several symptoms	0 (00%)	3 (37.5%)
2- BIOLOGY		
CRP at recovery (mg/l) ** (n = 12 cases)	192.5 (120-300)	155.93 (95.5-384)
White blood cell count	13107.5 (6630-17700)	14606.25 (8400-25500)

Table 10: Comparison of preoperative clinical and laboratory data (PPO) between the Discharged and Deceased groups (n = 12)

Features	Leavers (n = 04)	Deceased (n = 08)
-Time between discovery and recovery		
Not included	0 (00%)	1(12.5%)
0 day	0 (00%)	4 (50%)
1 day	2 (50%)	0 (00%)
2 days	0 (00%)	2 (25%)
3 days	1 (25%)	0 (00%)
More than 3 days	1 (25%)	1 (12.5%)

Table 11: Comparison of time between discovery and recovery in the Discharged and Deceased groups (n = 12)

Features	Leavers (n = 04)	Deceased (n = 08)
-Causes of PPO		
Releasing the anastomosis	3 (75%)	4 (50%)
Disinsertion of drain	0 (00%)	1 (12.5%)
Aberrant channel	0 (00%)	1 (12.5%)
Perforation of an organ	1 (25%)	1 (12.5%)
Suture loosening	0 (00%)	1 (12.5%)

Table 12: Comparison of data on causes of PPO between the

Discharged and Deceased groups (n = 12)

Features	Leavers (n = 04)	Deceased (n = 08)
- Antibiotic therapy used		
Monotherapy	0 (00)	1 (12.5)
Dual therapy	1 (25)	5 (62.5)
Tritherapy	3 (75)	2 (25)

Table 13: Comparison of data on Antibiotic Therapy Used throughout

the period of hospitalisation in the intensive care unit between the

Discharged and Deceased groups (n = 12)

V.DISCUSSION

1. Comprehensive descriptive study (epidemiology, diagnosis and treatment)

If we compare the global data with those from our study, we find a slight difference in the results.

The mean age is estimated at 53.3 years with a variation between 37 and 58 years in the different studies with **a sex ratio** of 1.2 with a variation between 0.5 and 1.8 (in **our sample the mean age is 62.25 with a sex ratio of 1.4**), which means that the incidence is almost the same between women and men regardless of the sample and the country studied. However, the age of onset in our country is high compared with samples from other countries.

The most frequent **sign of discovery** in the various studies was fever, with a percentage varying between 9% and 74%, followed by abdominal pain varying between 21 and 66% (**in our sample, the most frequent symptom was abdominal pain at 34%**) with **a diagnosis time** of 7.3 days (**in our sample it was 4.67 days**)

Antibiotic therapy in the case of PPO is much more probabilistic due to the failure to identify the germ at the time of the initial operation, and in the post-intervention period, we note that the use of **dual therapy** is the most frequent, with a variation of between 7 and 85%, with a percentage of 50% in our sample. Montravers implicated inappropriate bi-antibiotic therapy in the occurrence of complications after re-operation, in 50% of cases : Antibiotic therapy would therefore have an impact on the morbi-mortality of the patient with PPO.In our study, **anastomotic loosening** was **the main cause of**

PPO, with a percentage of 58.3% (in the other studies it varied between 46 and 68%). **The cause of PPO was the same in all the samples studied**.

2. Mortality

Prognosis depends on the speed with which the diagnosis is made and the effectiveness of the treatment administered. For Koperna and Schulz, only a rapid decision to re-explore within the first 48 hours following diagnosis can reduce mortality. Bohnenet al report a mortality rate of 35% in the case of early re-exploration, compared with 65% in the case of re-exploration more than 48 hours after diagnosis. late. Consequently, the occurrence of poly visceral failures or the appearance of a state of shock with no obvious origin will be formal criteria for reintervention. A white laparotomy is always less serious than a late repeat operation. Apart from this situation, the decision to repeat surgery will be based on a range of clinical and biological arguments supported by morphological data.

Mortality varies from study to study, ranging from 35 to 60% (in our sample it is estimated at 66.7%).

3.4. Prevention of postoperative peritonitis

The prevention of PPO is based on the control of FDR and appropriate treatment as quickly as possible.

VI. RESOURCES

• Preparing patients

- Psychic :

Information for patients on all stages of the procedure, risks and post-operative follow-up (especially in the case of digestive neoplasia).

- Body :

A suitable diet to promote healing and combat malnutrition (which can lead to anastomosis loosening), weight loss and regular physical activity before scheduled operations.

- History and co-morbidities :

Adaptation of treatments used for associated pathologies (hypertension, diabetes, heart disease) and regular monitoring of these therapeutic prescriptions to achieve these therapeutic objectives.

• The initial intervention

It is very important to adapt the initial surgical procedure and to favour **2-stage surgery,** especially for digestive neoplasia, to avoid the risk of loosening, which is the most frequent cause.

Approach: favour laparoscopic procedures and avoid laparotomies as much as possible (risk of infection is much higher).

• Post-operative follow-up

- Intensive care unit care

- Regular clinical and biological monitoring and investigation of the slightest doubt as early as possible (white laparotomy is less harmful to the patient than late intervention).

- Use of tritherapies (ATB) is more effective (where it has been noted that 75% of patients discharged are on tritherapy) and adapt TRT as quickly as possible depending on the germ involved

- Controlling the source of infection

VII. CONCLUSION

PPOs are emergencies that are often difficult to diagnose (in the postoperative period) and are treated medico-surgically, with a generally poor prognosis, particularly in frail patients or those treated late. Early diagnosis and treatment are the cornerstones of care. "It is therefore essential to take a precautionary approach, bearing in mind that a white laparotomy is less invasive than a white laparotomy. deleterious for the patient than late intervention".

Management algorithm

Therapeutic management is **multidisciplinary, involving the** intensive care anaesthetist, surgeon, radiologist and microbiologist. It includes rapid and optimal haemodynamic resuscitation, probabilistic antibiotic therapy chosen according to the bacteriological profile of the hospital and the nosocomial nature of the infection and adapted to the antibiogram, and the most perfect surgical procedure possible.

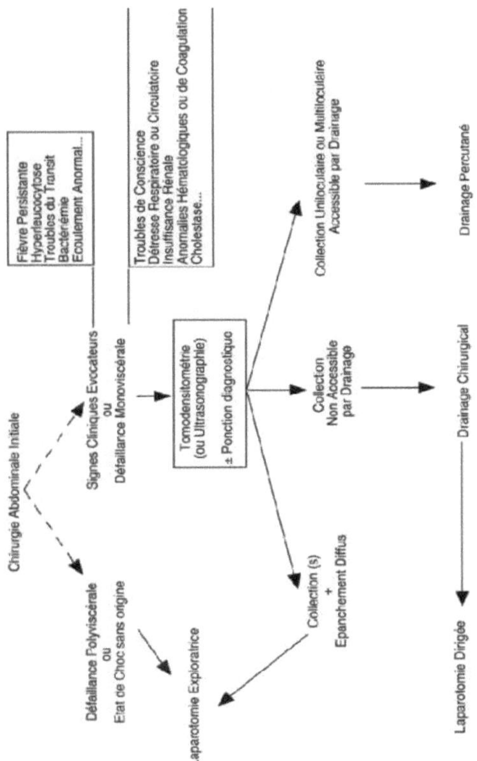

Figure 11: The decision tree in the event of abnormal evolution at following abdominal surgery.

VIII. SUMMARIES

Title : **Postoperative peritonitis in the intensive care unit**

Author : **GUEZGOUZ MOHAMED**

**BENTOUNES FATIHA MOHAMADIA FARAADJ BOUABAIA
SOUAD CHAHRAZED.**

Supervisor :**Pr SOUMIA BENBERNOU**

Key word : Postoperative peritonitis - Risk factors - Neoplasia

– Digestive surgery - Mortality.

● **Introduction** :

Postoperative peritonitis is a serious infection that occurs after abdomino-pelvic surgery, most often digestive surgery. The aim of this study was :

- Determine the general risk factors for postoperative peritonitis?
- Keeping track of changes in patients' general condition?

- What is the incidence and what are the predictive risk factors for mortality in postoperative peritonitis (i.e. poor prognosis risk factors)?
- How can postoperative peritonitis be prevented?

● **Methodology** :

This is a retrospective cohort study of cases who had postoperative peritonitis between 10 September 2022 and 11 February 2023 (05 months) at the Mostaganem University Hospital. The parameters studied were demographic, diagnostic, therapeutic and prognostic. The primary outcome was death or discharge from the intensive care unit. We compared the group of patients discharged and those who died in terms of these parameters.

- **Results** :

12 patients were included in the study. The mean age of our patients was 62.25, with a clear male predominance (sex ratio M/F equal to 1.4). The overall mortality rate was 66.7%.

- **Conclusion**:

Post-operative peritonitis is a serious diagnostic and therapeutic emergency. Diagnosis is often difficult (postoperative period). Treatment is medico-surgical. Mortality due to postoperative peritonitis remains a major problem The prognosis could be poor, particularly in frail patients or those treated late.

BIBLIOGRAPHY

- **Books**

1. Kb gastroenterology

2. KB resuscitation

2. Gastroenterology codex

3. **Martingal gastroenterology**

- **Websites 1.PubMed**

2. https://www.bibliosante.ml/bitstream/handle/123456789/3756/19M4
32.pdf;jsessionid=A8FAC0246D50A6FA812D92699451FB87?seque
nce=1

3. https://www.ncbi.nlm.nih.gov/pmc/articles/PMC9883798/

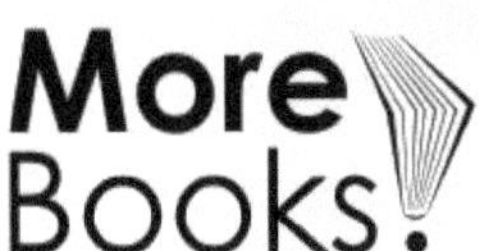

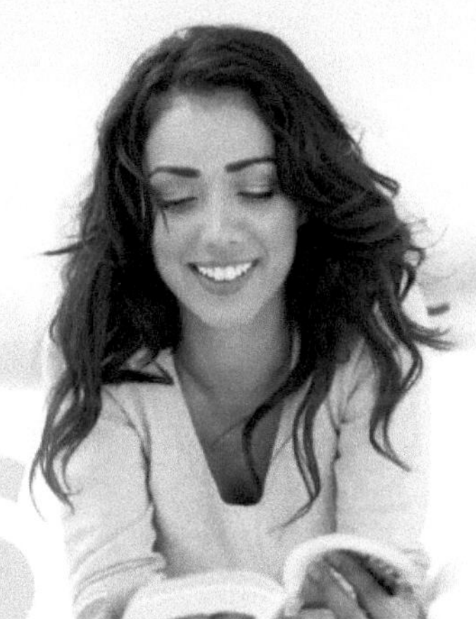

yes
I want morebooks!

Buy your books fast and straightforward online - at one of world's fastest growing online book stores! Environmentally sound due to Print-on-Demand technologies.

Buy your books online at
www.morebooks.shop

Kaufen Sie Ihre Bücher schnell und unkompliziert online – auf einer der am schnellsten wachsenden Buchhandelsplattformen weltweit! Dank Print-On-Demand umwelt- und ressourcenschonend produziert.

Bücher schneller online kaufen
www.morebooks.shop

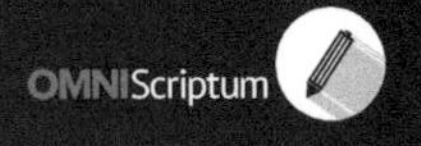

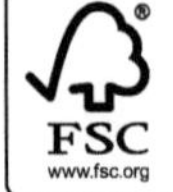
MIX
Papier aus verantwortungsvollen Quellen
Paper from responsible sources
FSC® C105338
FSC
www.fsc.org

Printed by Books on Demand GmbH, Norderstedt / Germany